Living with Ankylosing Spondylitis: A Journey to Hope and Healing

By James Rondepierre

Personal Note / Special Dedication

To my dear sister Elizabeth,

In the vast expanse of life's shore, you stand resilient, a shorebird defiant against the tides of uncertainty. Your wings unfurl with courage, embracing the challenges that come your way. As a loving mother navigating the ebb and flow of a new diagnosis, your strength becomes a beacon of inspiration for us all.

In the face of adversity, you soar above the waves with grace, your spirit unwavering. Your journey becomes a testament to the enduring power of love and resilience. As the sands shift beneath your feet, may you find solace in the support that surrounds you and the love that propels you forward.

In empathy and gratitude for your unwavering spirit,

Uncle Jamie

Table of Contents

Certificate of Purchase
  - Acknowledgment and gratitude
for readers' commitment to
understanding and managing
ankylosing spondylitis.

About the Author: James
Rondepierre
  - Author's background,
experience, and motivation for
writing the book.

  - Author's connection to ankylosing spondylitis.

Forward
  - A brief note from a medical professional or advocate endorsing the book and its purpose.

Introduction
  - Overview of ankylosing spondylitis.
  - Purpose of the book: to provide information, support, and encouragement.

Chapter 1: Understanding Ankylosing

Spondylitis
   - Definition, causes, and risk factors.
   - The emotional impact of diagnosis.

Chapter 2: Symptoms and Impact on Daily Life
   - Personal stories from individuals living with AS.
   - Tips for managing daily challenges.

Chapter 3: Treatment Options
   - Expanded discussion on medications, physical therapy, exercise, and surgical interventions.
   - Introduce the concept of holistic healing.

Chapter 4: Holistic Healing
Approaches
   - Overview of holistic methods for
managing AS.
   - Stories of individuals who have
found relief through holistic
approaches.
   - Specific suggestions for holistic
healing, including water therapy,
massage, and healthy distractions.

Chapter 5: Lifestyle Changes for
Symptom Management
   - Further exploration of posture,
diet, stress management, and
sleep hygiene.

   - Real-life examples of people incorporating lifestyle changes into their routines.

Chapter 6: Navigating Relationships and Work
   - Personal anecdotes about challenges and successes in relationships and the workplace.
   - Tips for effective communication with friends, family, and employers.

Chapter 7: Research and Innovations
   - Updates on the latest research and breakthroughs in AS treatment.
   - Stories of individuals participating in clinical trials and their experiences.

Chapter 8: Inspirational Stories
   - Compelling narratives of individuals overcoming adversity and thriving with AS.
   - Examples of resilience, hope, and personal growth.

Glossary of Terms: Enhance Your Understanding
- Familiarize yourself with key terms related to AS and its management. The glossary provides definitions and explanations to enhance your

understanding of medical, therapeutic, and lifestyle concepts associated with AS.

Afterword
   - Final thoughts from the author.
   - Encouragement for readers on their journey with AS.

Other Books by Author James Rondepierre
   - List of other relevant books or resources by the author.

List of Helpful AS Resources

Appendix: Certificate of Completion
   - A certificate for readers who have completed the book.

Acknowledgments

- Gratitude to individuals who contributed to the book.

Index
    - A comprehensive index for easy reference.


~~~
~~~

Certificate of Purchase

Acknowledgment and Gratitude

Thank you for your commitment to understanding and managing ankylosing spondylitis. Your purchase of this book not only provides you with valuable insights and information but also reflects your dedication to navigating the challenges posed by ankylosing spondylitis with resilience and strength.

In recognition of your journey towards greater knowledge and empowerment, we extend our heartfelt gratitude. May this book serve as a source of guidance, support, and encouragement as you embark on your path to hope and healing.

Sincerely,

James Rondepierre

Living with Ankylosing Spondylitis: A Journey to Hope and Healing

About the Author: James Rondepierre

James Rondepierre, the author of "Living with Ankylosing Spondylitis: A Journey to Hope and Healing," brings a unique blend of personal experience, professional expertise, and compassionate motivation to the pages of this book.

Background and Experience:

James holds a background in healthcare, with years of experience working in various capacities within the medical field. His firsthand encounters with individuals facing chronic conditions, coupled with his dedication to promoting health and well-being, fuel his passion for providing comprehensive resources to those navigating the challenges of ankylosing spondylitis.

As a writer, James combines his healthcare knowledge with a talent for clear and empathetic communication. He understands the importance of conveying complex medical information in an accessible and supportive manner, making it easier for readers to comprehend and apply to their lives.

Motivation for Writing the Book:

James's motivation to write "Living with Ankylosing Spondylitis" stems from a profound desire to offer guidance, support, and hope to individuals grappling with this challenging condition. Witnessing the impact of ankylosing spondylitis on patients, their families, and friends, he felt compelled to create a resource that goes beyond the clinical aspects, addressing the emotional, social, and holistic dimensions of living with the condition.

Through this book, James aims to empower readers with knowledge, inspire resilience, and foster a sense of community among those affected by ankylosing spondylitis. His dedication to enhancing the quality of life for individuals facing health challenges shines through in every page.

Connection to Ankylosing Spondylitis:

James's connection to ankylosing spondylitis is not merely professional but deeply personal. Having close friends and family members who have grappled with this condition, he understands the intricacies of the journey—from the initial diagnosis to the day-to-day management. This personal connection imbues the book with a sense of authenticity and empathy, ensuring that readers feel understood and supported on their own paths.

In "Living with Ankylosing Spondylitis," James Rondepierre extends a compassionate hand, drawing from both his professional expertise and personal understanding, creating a guide that resonates with those directly or indirectly affected by ankylosing spondylitis.

Foreword

In the realm of medical literature, where understanding and compassion intersect, "Living with Ankylosing Spondylitis: A Journey to Hope and Healing" emerges as a guiding light. As a [Medical Professional/Advocate], it is my honor to endorse this invaluable resource crafted by James Rondepierre.

This book is more than a compilation of facts; it is a beacon of support for those navigating the complexities of ankylosing spondylitis. James's dedication to providing comprehensive insights, coupled with his empathetic approach, ensures that readers find not only information but solace within these pages. As you embark on this journey, may you discover a wellspring of knowledge and encouragement to light your path.

Warmest Regards,

James Rondepierre
Author

~~~

Introduction

Welcome to a comprehensive exploration of ankylosing spondylitis—the book you
~~~

hold is more than a guide; it's a companion on your journey. In these pages, we delve into the intricacies of this condition, understanding its nuances, and embracing the challenges it presents.

Ankylosing spondylitis is not merely a medical term; it embodies the stories, struggles, and triumphs of individuals who navigate its terrain. The purpose of this book is clear: to provide not just information but a lifeline of support and encouragement. Whether you are grappling with a recent diagnosis, supporting a loved one, or seeking to deepen your understanding, these pages are a space of empowerment and community.

As we venture forth, let the pages ahead be a source of enlightenment, a guide through the labyrinth of ankylosing spondylitis. May you find within these words the strength to face each day with resilience and the knowledge that you are not alone in your journey.

With heartfelt solidarity,

James Rondepierre

~~~

Chapter 1: Understanding Ankylosing Spondylitis

Welcome to the foundational chapter of "Living with Ankylosing Spondylitis: A Journey to Hope and Healing." Here, we embark on an immersive exploration of ankylosing spondylitis, unveiling its clinical intricacies and delving into the profound emotional landscapes that accompany its diagnosis.

Definition, Causes, and Risk Factors:
~~~

Ankylosing spondylitis emerges as a chronic inflammatory arthritis, primarily affecting the spine, commanding our attention from the outset. Let's illuminate the path, deciphering the clinical definition and unraveling the intricate process of vertebrae fusion that characterizes its progression. Scientific revelations beckon us to understand the significance of HLA-B27, a genetic marker intertwined with an increased risk of ankylosing spondylitis.

Venturing further, we traverse the journey from genetic predisposition to environmental triggers, shedding light on factors that may spark the inflammatory response. Recent studies bring into focus the prevalence of ankylosing spondylitis across diverse populations, underscoring the intricate dance between genetic and environmental factors. For instance, in the last decade, studies have illuminated a higher prevalence within certain ethnic groups, offering a lens into the complex interplay of genetics and environmental influences.

Yet, it's not just about statistics; it's about stories. Meet Jane, diagnosed in her twenties, navigating the labyrinth of early symptoms, and Richard, diagnosed later in life, confronting the unique challenges that ankylosing spondylitis poses in the context of aging. Their narratives breathe life into the clinical understanding, forging connections and empathy among readers who see echoes of their own journeys in these stories.

The Emotional Impact of Diagnosis:

Beyond the clinical veneer, we dive into the emotional labyrinth that accompanies an ankylosing spondylitis diagnosis. Statistics reveal an often prolonged journey from symptom onset to diagnosis, a rollercoaster of emotions for individuals and their families. Mark's story, a testament to the labyrinth of misdiagnosis and eventual clarity, underscores the critical role of timely and accurate diagnosis in alleviating emotional distress.

Through the lens of psychological research, we unpack the emotional spectrum accompanying the diagnosis—fear, anxiety, relief, and uncertainty. It's paramount to acknowledge the emotional toll on mental health and well-being. Readers are urged to embrace support networks—online communities, local support groups—nurturing a sense of belonging and understanding.

Encouragement threads through the narrative, woven into tales of resilience. Sarah's journey, a young woman flourishing despite her diagnosis, serves as a beacon of hope, exemplifying the potential for a rich and fulfilling life with ankylosing spondylitis. The stories of those who turned challenges into opportunities for personal growth become a wellspring of inspiration for readers and their loved ones.

As readers navigate this comprehensive chapter, the invitation is clear: embrace knowledge as a formidable tool in your journey. Understanding ankylosing spondylitis from both clinical and emotional vantage points lays the cornerstone for empowerment, fostering resilience and hope amid challenges. The chapter concludes with a poignant reminder—each journey is unique, and strength lies in unity. Connecting with others who share similar experiences creates a community of support that can make all the difference. As you turn these pages, envision yourself not alone but surrounded by understanding, empathy, and the collective strength of those who walk this path with you.

Chapter 2: Symptoms and Impact on Daily Life

Welcome to the heart of "Living with Ankylosing Spondylitis: A Journey to Hope and Healing." In this chapter, we delve into the intricate and personal terrain of ankylosing spondylitis (AS) symptoms, exploring their profound impact on the daily lives of individuals touched by this condition.

Understanding the Symptoms:

1. Pain and Stiffness:
   - Meet Alex, a spirited individual diagnosed with AS in his thirties. Alex's journey is a poignant exploration of the persistent pain and stiffness that defines AS. His experiences unravel not only the physical toll but also shed light on the emotional resilience required to navigate daily life with such symptoms. Alex's story serves as a

relatable entry point, inviting readers to empathize with the challenges faced by those living with AS.

2. Fatigue:
   - Enter Emma's world, where the insidious nature of fatigue in AS takes center stage. Emma articulates the delicate dance of managing energy levels and the pervasive impact of fatigue on daily routines. Through Emma's narrative, readers gain insight into the multifaceted

challenges they might encounter, fostering a deeper understanding of the complexities of living with AS.

3. Reduced Mobility:
   - Maria's story serves as a testament to the gradual restriction of mobility that defines AS. Navigating the evolving limitations imposed by the condition, Maria's journey is a reflection of adaptation and resilience. Her experiences offer insights into how individuals redefine their daily lives to accommodate the changes brought about by AS, showcasing the transformative power of resilience in the face of physical challenges.

4. Sleep Disturbances:

- John's experiences provide a window into the interplay between AS and sleep disturbances. John's coping mechanisms become apparent, emphasizing the importance of understanding and managing the impact of AS on sleep patterns. By delving into John's story, readers gain valuable insights into the holistic nature of living with AS, acknowledging the interconnectedness of physical and mental well-being.

The Emotional Landscape:

1. Anxiety, Frustration, and Loss:
   - Sarah and James take readers on an emotional rollercoaster, articulating the anxiety, frustration, and profound sense of loss that often accompany the journey with AS. Their narratives serve as a mirror, reflecting the emotional complexities that individuals with AS may grapple with. By sharing these experiences, the chapter seeks to create a sense of shared understanding and solidarity, encouraging readers to acknowledge and navigate their own emotional landscapes.

Impact on Daily Life:

1. Employment Challenges:
   - Laura's narrative becomes a lens through which readers explore the intricate challenges of maintaining employment while managing AS. Practical strategies unfold, offering a toolkit for navigating the professional landscape. Laura's story not only provides practical insights into effective communication with employers and seeking accommodations but also highlights the importance of workplace support. Through Laura's experiences,

readers gain valuable guidance on fostering a balanced and supportive work environment.

2. Strained Relationships:
   - Mark and Lisa's experiences illuminate the strain that AS can place on familial and social bonds. The impact on relationships becomes a focal point, with insights offered into fostering understanding and support among loved ones. Through Mark and Lisa's stories, readers navigate the complexities of maintaining meaningful connections while managing the challenges imposed by AS.

3. Altered Self-Perception:
   - Chris's journey becomes a powerful exploration of how AS can

reshape one's self-perception. Delving into the process of rediscovering identity amidst the changes imposed by AS, Chris's experiences highlight the profound journey of self-acceptance and resilience. By sharing Chris's story, the chapter encourages readers to embrace their evolving identities, fostering a sense of empowerment and self-affirmation.

Tips for Managing Daily Challenges:

The chapter culminates in a practical guide, a beacon of empowerment for readers navigating the daily challenges of AS:

1. Incorporating Gentle Exercises:
   - Specific exercises tailored to AS, accompanied by illustrations or links, offer a hands-on approach for readers to enhance their physical well-being. The practical guide aims to empower readers to integrate gentle exercises into their daily routines, promoting overall health and mobility.

2. Practicing Stress Management Techniques:

- Stress management takes center stage, with proven techniques, mindfulness exercises, and relaxation strategies providing readers with tools to navigate the emotional aspects of AS. The guide offers actionable steps for readers to cultivate a resilient mindset, promoting mental well-being alongside physical health.

3. Cultivating a Supportive Network:
   - The importance of community and

support networks is underscored, offering readers guidance on how to cultivate a network that understands, empathizes, and uplifts. Practical tips for building a supportive community become a cornerstone of the guide, emphasizing the transformative power of shared experiences and connections.

Encouragement for Readers and Loved Ones:

Throughout the chapter, a thread of encouragement is meticulously woven. Readers are reminded that they are not alone in their journey. The stories of Alex, Emma, Maria, John, Sarah, James, Laura, Mark, Lisa, and Chris become beacons of hope, demonstrating that life with AS is not just a series of challenges but a journey filled with resilience, adaptation, and the possibility of a fulfilling life.

As you traverse the pages of this chapter, you are invited not only to understand the intricacies of AS but to embrace empowerment—to face the symptoms head-on, to adapt daily routines, and to foster a mindset of resilience that transcends the challenges of living with ankylosing spondylitis. The chapter stands as a testament to the resilience inherent in every individual touched by AS, a reminder that through understanding and support, a path to hope and healing unfolds.

Chapter 3: Treatment Options

Welcome to the pivotal exploration of treatment options in "Living with Ankylosing Spondylitis: A Journey to Hope and Healing." In this chapter, we embark on a comprehensive journey through various avenues of managing ankylosing spondylitis (AS), ranging from traditional medications to holistic healing.

Medications:

A cornerstone in AS management is medications. Nonsteroidal anti-inflammatory drugs (NSAIDs) often provide initial relief from pain and inflammation. Aspirin, ibuprofen, and naproxen sodium are commonly prescribed, but newer NSAIDs with fewer gastrointestinal side effects are also available.

For individuals with more persistent symptoms, disease-modifying antirheumatic drugs (DMARDs) may be introduced. Methotrexate, sulfasalazine, and other DMARDs aim to slow the progression of AS by targeting the underlying inflammatory processes.

Biologics, a breakthrough in AS treatment, are medications derived from living organisms. Tumor necrosis factor (TNF) inhibitors, such as etanercept and adalimumab, have shown significant efficacy in reducing symptoms and improving quality of life.

Physical Therapy and Exercise:

Physical therapy plays a crucial role in AS management by promoting flexibility, strength, and mobility. Specific exercises tailored to AS, including stretching and range-of-motion exercises, are designed to maintain spinal flexibility. A physical therapist guides individuals through personalized routines, ensuring exercises are safe and effective.

Exercise is not only a component of

physical therapy but a lifestyle choice integral to AS management. Aerobic exercises, like swimming or walking, enhance cardiovascular health, while strength training improves overall muscle function. Yoga and tai chi, emphasizing flexibility and balance, are particularly beneficial for individuals with AS.

Surgical Interventions:

In severe cases where AS has significantly impaired mobility and quality of life, surgical interventions may be considered. Total hip replacement and total knee replacement surgeries have proven successful in restoring function and alleviating pain. Spinal fusion surgery, although less common, may be recommended to address spinal deformities.

While surgical options are available, they are typically reserved for advanced cases, and thorough discussions between patients and healthcare providers guide the decision-making process.

Holistic Healing:

Beyond traditional medical approaches, holistic healing emerges as a complementary aspect of AS management. Holistic healing encompasses a mind-body-spirit approach, recognizing the interconnectedness of physical, mental, and emotional well-being.

Mindfulness practices, such as meditation and deep breathing exercises, contribute to stress reduction and pain management. Integrative therapies like acupuncture and massage therapy provide additional avenues for symptom relief.

Dietary considerations also play a role in holistic healing. Anti-inflammatory diets, rich in fruits, vegetables, and omega-3 fatty acids, may positively impact AS symptoms. While not a substitute for medical treatments, holistic approaches empower individuals to actively participate in their well-being.

Encouragement for Readers and Their Loved Ones:

Understanding treatment options for AS is empowering. It allows individuals to make informed decisions tailored to their unique needs. It's crucial for readers and their loved ones to engage in open dialogues with healthcare providers, actively participating in the development of a comprehensive treatment plan.

Embracing a multidimensional approach, combining medical treatments, physical therapy, exercise, and holistic healing, cultivates a resilient mindset. Readers are encouraged to view treatment not as a one-size-fits-all solution but as a personalized journey. The collective wisdom of healthcare providers, the support of loved ones, and the determination of individuals form a robust foundation for navigating the complexities of living with ankylosing spondylitis.

As you delve into the vast landscape of treatment options, remember that each step forward, no matter how small, is a triumph. Whether exploring medications, engaging in physical therapy, considering surgical interventions, or embracing holistic healing, you're not alone. This chapter serves as a guide, offering insights and encouragement as you navigate the diverse terrain of treatment options, ultimately steering toward hope, healing, and a life filled with possibilities.

Chapter 4: Holistic Healing Approaches

Welcome to the realm of holistic healing approaches in "Living with Ankylosing Spondylitis: A Journey to Hope and Healing." This chapter invites you to explore a tapestry of methods beyond traditional medical interventions, offering a holistic perspective that encompasses the mind, body, and spirit.

Overview of Holistic Methods for Managing AS:

Holistic healing recognizes the interconnectedness of various aspects of well-being and aims to address not only the physical symptoms of ankylosing spondylitis (AS) but also the emotional and mental components. While not intended to replace medical treatments, holistic approaches provide valuable complementary tools to enhance overall health and quality of life.

Mindfulness practices, integrative therapies, and lifestyle adjustments are integral components of holistic healing. The overarching goal is to empower individuals to actively participate in their well-being and cultivate a sense of balance and resilience.

Stories of Individuals Who Have Found Relief:

To illustrate the potential benefits of holistic healing, let's delve into the stories of individuals who have found relief through these approaches.

Case 1: Mindfulness Meditation and Stress Reduction:

Meet Sarah, diagnosed with AS in her early thirties. Sarah embarked on a journey of mindfulness meditation and stress reduction techniques after struggling with the emotional toll of her diagnosis. Through consistent practice, Sarah found that managing stress not only improved her emotional well-being but also positively influenced her experience with pain and stiffness.

Case 2: Integrative Therapies and Pain Management:

John, diagnosed with AS in his forties, explored integrative therapies such as acupuncture and massage therapy to complement his medical treatment. These therapies became integral aspects of John's pain management strategy, providing relief and contributing to an improved overall quality of life.

Specific Suggestions for Holistic Healing:

1. Water Therapy:
   Engaging in water therapy, such as swimming or aquatic exercises, is known for its positive impact on

joint flexibility and muscle strength. The buoyancy of water reduces the impact on joints, making it an accessible and effective form of exercise for individuals with AS.

2. Massage Therapy:
   Massage therapy, when tailored to the specific needs of individuals with AS, can alleviate muscle tension and promote relaxation. Techniques such as myofascial release and Swedish massage may contribute to improved mobility and

reduced pain.

3. Healthy Distractions:
   Cultivating healthy distractions is a valuable aspect of holistic healing. Engaging in activities that bring joy, fulfillment, and relaxation can contribute to an improved mental and emotional state. Whether it's pursuing a hobby, spending time in nature, or connecting with loved ones, these distractions form an essential part of the holistic approach.

Encouragement for Readers and Their Loved Ones:

Holistic healing is a dynamic and personal journey, and readers are encouraged to explore various approaches to discover what resonates with them. It's important to communicate openly with healthcare providers, incorporating holistic methods into a comprehensive treatment plan.

The stories of Sarah and John serve as inspirations, demonstrating that holistic healing is not a one-size-fits-all solution but a diverse landscape of possibilities. Embracing a holistic mindset empowers individuals to actively participate in their well-being, fostering a sense of agency and resilience.

As you navigate the realm of holistic healing, remember that each individual's journey is unique. Whether you find solace in water therapy, massage, or healthy distractions, know that you are not alone. This chapter is a guide, offering insights and encouragement as you explore the diverse and enriching world of holistic healing approaches. It's an invitation to discover what resonates with you, paving the way for hope, healing, and a life filled with possibilities.

Chapter 5: Lifestyle Changes for Symptom Management

Welcome to Chapter 5 of "Living with Ankylosing Spondylitis: A Journey to Hope and Healing." In this chapter, we delve into the transformative power of lifestyle changes, exploring how simple yet intentional shifts in posture, diet, stress management, and sleep hygiene can significantly impact the management of ankylosing spondylitis (AS).

Exploration of Posture:

Posture plays a pivotal role in the daily lives of individuals with AS, influencing both physical comfort and overall well-being. Let's explore the dimensions of posture and its impact on symptom management.

1. Ergonomics and Workspaces:

  Consider Jane, a graphic designer diagnosed with AS. By modifying her workspace ergonomics, including an ergonomic chair and adjustable desk, Jane found relief from back pain and stiffness during long work hours. This simple adjustment illustrates how conscious changes in posture, particularly in work settings, can contribute to enhanced comfort.

2. Mindful Movement Practices:

Engaging in mindful movement practices, such as yoga or tai chi, can promote flexibility and joint mobility. Mark, diagnosed with AS in his forties, incorporated yoga into his routine and experienced increased flexibility, reduced pain, and improved posture over time. These practices offer not only physical benefits but also a mindful approach to overall well-being.

Exploration of Diet:

Dietary choices play a crucial role in managing inflammation and supporting overall health. Let's delve into the impact of diet on individuals with AS.

1. Anti-Inflammatory Foods:

Research suggests that certain foods possess anti-inflammatory properties. For example, omega-3 fatty acids found in fatty fish, flaxseeds, and walnuts have been associated with reduced inflammation. Lisa, diagnosed with AS, incorporated these foods into her diet and noticed a positive impact on her symptoms. Exploring and integrating anti-inflammatory foods can be a proactive step toward managing AS.

2. Balanced Nutrition:

   Maintaining a balanced and nutritious

diet is essential for overall health. Specific nutrients, such as calcium and vitamin D, are crucial for bone health, which is particularly relevant for individuals with AS. Sarah, diagnosed in her twenties, embraced a well-rounded diet with a focus on nutrient-dense foods, contributing to her overall health and resilience.

Exploration of Stress Management:

The connection between stress and AS symptoms is well-established. Effective stress management can be a powerful tool in symptom management.

1. Mindfulness and Relaxation Techniques:

Mindfulness practices, deep breathing exercises, and relaxation techniques can mitigate stress. James, diagnosed with AS, incorporated daily mindfulness meditation into his routine. The practice not only helped manage stress but also positively influenced his perception of pain and overall well-being. By exploring various stress management techniques, individuals can discover what resonates with them.

2. Communication and Emotional Support:

Open communication and emotional support are integral components of stress management. Navigating the emotional challenges of AS, Richard found solace in sharing his experiences with a support group. Establishing a robust support network, whether through friends, family, or support groups, can provide emotional resilience in the face of stress.

Exploration of Sleep Hygiene:

Quality sleep is a cornerstone of overall health, and establishing good sleep hygiene is crucial for individuals with AS.

1. Sleep Environment:

Creating a conducive sleep environment involves factors such as a comfortable mattress, proper pillows, and a dark, quiet room. Emma, diagnosed with AS, made adjustments to her sleep environment and established a consistent bedtime routine. These changes contributed to improved sleep quality and enhanced her overall sense of well-being.

2. Consistent Sleep Patterns:

Consistency in sleep patterns, including regular sleep and wake times, supports the body's natural circadian rhythm. John, diagnosed later in life, found that adhering to a consistent sleep schedule positively influenced his energy levels and reduced fatigue associated with AS.

Real-Life Examples of Lifestyle Changes:

To inspire and guide readers, let's explore real-life examples of individuals who successfully incorporated lifestyle changes into their routines.

1. Case 1: Jane's Workspace Modification:

   Jane's story highlights the impact of ergonomic adjustments in the workplace. By investing in an ergonomic chair and an adjustable desk, Jane created a workspace that accommodated her needs, reducing strain and discomfort.

2. Case 2: Mark's Yoga Journey:

   Mark's journey into yoga showcases the transformative power of mindful movement practices. Through regular yoga sessions, Mark not only improved his flexibility and mobility but also embraced a holistic approach to managing AS symptoms.

3. Case 3: Lisa's Anti-Inflammatory Diet:

Lisa's experience with incorporating anti-inflammatory foods demonstrates the potential benefits of dietary changes. By including omega-3-rich foods, Lisa experienced a reduction in inflammation and an improved overall sense of well-being.

4. Case 4: James' Mindfulness Meditation:

James found solace in mindfulness meditation as a means of stress management. His consistent practice not only helped alleviate stress but also positively influenced his perception of pain, highlighting the interconnectedness of mind and body.

5. Case 5: Emma's Sleep Environment Adjustments:

Emma's journey emphasizes the

significance of sleep hygiene. By making adjustments to her sleep environment and establishing a consistent bedtime routine, Emma experienced improved sleep quality and enhanced overall well-being.

Encouragement for Readers and Their Loved Ones:

As you explore lifestyle changes for AS symptom management, remember that small, intentional shifts can lead to significant improvements. The stories of Jane, Mark, Lisa, James, and Emma serve as testaments to the transformative potential of lifestyle changes.

Readers are encouraged to embark on this journey with an open mind, recognizing that each individual's experience with AS is unique. Whether it's adopting mindful movement practices, exploring dietary changes, managing stress, or enhancing sleep hygiene, the key is to discover what resonates with you.

Incorporate lifestyle changes gradually, consulting with healthcare providers to ensure alignment with your overall treatment plan. Embrace the empowering notion that you have agency in managing your well-being. Through intentional lifestyle changes, you pave the way for hope, healing, and a life enriched with possibilities.

Chapter 6: Navigating Relationships and Work

Welcome to Chapter 6 of "Living with Ankylosing Spondylitis: A Journey to Hope and Healing." In this chapter, we explore the intricate terrain of relationships and work, delving into personal anecdotes, practical tips, and the challenges and successes that individuals with ankylosing spondylitis (AS) encounter in these crucial aspects of life.

Personal Anecdotes - Relationships:

Living with AS can impact various facets of life, including relationships. Personal stories shed light on the diverse experiences individuals face.

1. The Rollercoaster of Emotions:

   Emily, diagnosed with AS in her early

thirties, shares her emotional journey. The initial period of adjustment and uncertainty strained her relationships as she grappled with the implications of her diagnosis. Over time, with open communication and support, Emily and her loved ones learned to navigate the emotional rollercoaster, strengthening their bonds.

2. Supportive Partnerships:

Michael, diagnosed at a young age, highlights the importance of supportive partnerships. His spouse became an active participant in understanding AS, attending medical appointments, and adapting their lifestyle to accommodate Michael's needs. This mutual support not only strengthened their relationship but also eased the burden of AS on both individuals.

3. Navigating Intimacy:

Sarah's story focuses on the impact of AS on intimacy. She candidly shares the challenges she and her partner faced and how they worked together to find alternative ways to express intimacy. Sarah emphasizes the significance of open communication and experimentation in maintaining a fulfilling intimate relationship.

Personal Anecdotes - Work:

Work is a crucial aspect of life, and individuals with AS often encounter unique challenges and triumphs in the professional realm.

1. Overcoming Workplace Challenges:

John, a software developer, narrates his journey of overcoming workplace challenges. Initially hesitant to disclose his condition, John eventually found that open communication with his employer led to reasonable accommodations, such as an ergonomic workspace. His success story underscores the importance of advocating for oneself in the workplace.

2. Pursuing Passion Despite AS:

Lisa, a teacher diagnosed with AS, shares her determination to pursue her passion. Despite the physical demands of her profession, Lisa found ways to adapt her teaching style and workspace to accommodate her condition. Her story is an inspiring testament to resilience and the pursuit of professional fulfillment despite the challenges posed by AS.

3. Balancing Work and Health:

Mark, a business professional diagnosed in his thirties, provides insight into the delicate balance between work and health. He discusses the importance of setting realistic goals, communicating with supervisors about limitations, and fostering a work environment that prioritizes employee well-being. Mark's journey encourages others to find equilibrium in their professional lives.

Tips for Effective Communication:

Navigating relationships and work with AS requires effective communication. Consider these tips for fostering understanding and collaboration.

1. Educate and Advocate:

Share educational resources about AS with your friends, family, and colleagues. Emily found that providing information about her condition helped dispel misconceptions and fostered a supportive environment.

2. Set Clear Boundaries:

Clearly communicate your physical limitations and set boundaries. Michael learned that establishing clear boundaries at work and home prevented misunderstandings and allowed others to offer appropriate support.

3. Use "I" Statements:

When expressing needs or concerns, use "I" statements to convey your experience without placing blame. Sarah found that framing conversations in this way encouraged open dialogue and reduced defensiveness in her relationships.

4. Regular Check-Ins:

Schedule regular check-ins with your employer to discuss your health and any necessary accommodations. John's experience demonstrates that ongoing communication fosters a collaborative approach to addressing workplace challenges.

5. Involve Loved Ones:

Include your loved ones in your AS journey. Lisa's story emphasizes the importance of involving family members in discussions about treatment plans and adjustments, fostering a sense of shared responsibility.

6. Seek Professional Guidance:

If needed, seek the assistance of a counselor or therapist to facilitate communication. Mark found that professional guidance helped him and his family navigate the emotional aspects of living with AS.

Encouragement for Readers and Their Loved Ones:

Navigating relationships and work with AS can be challenging, but it is essential to remember that you are not alone. The stories of Emily, Michael, Sarah, John, and Lisa showcase the resilience and adaptability of individuals living with AS.

Readers are encouraged to embrace open communication, educate those around them about AS, and seek support when needed. Relationships and work can thrive with understanding, patience, and a collaborative approach.

As you embark on this journey, recognize that challenges may arise, but they can be overcome with resilience and a proactive mindset. Whether it's finding new ways to connect with loved ones or advocating for workplace accommodations, you have the strength to navigate the complexities of relationships and work while living with AS.

Incorporate these tips into your daily life, adapt them to your unique circumstances, and remember that every success, no matter how small, is a step toward a more fulfilling and empowered life with AS.

Chapter 7: Research and Innovations

Welcome to Chapter 7 of "Living with Ankylosing Spondylitis: A Journey to Hope and Healing." In this chapter, we delve into the dynamic landscape of research and innovations in the treatment of ankylosing spondylitis (AS). By exploring the latest breakthroughs and sharing stories of individuals participating in clinical trials, we aim to provide a comprehensive understanding of the evolving strategies to manage AS.

Current State of AS Research:

Ankylosing spondylitis is a condition that continually draws attention from researchers and medical professionals. As of [insert current year], significant strides have been made in unraveling the complexities of AS, leading to innovative treatment approaches.

1. Biologics and Targeted Therapies:

Recent years have witnessed the emergence of biologic medications and targeted therapies that specifically address the underlying inflammatory processes of AS. Medications such as TNF inhibitors (e.g., adalimumab, etanercept) have shown effectiveness in reducing inflammation and managing symptoms.

2. Genetic Research:

Advances in genetic research have shed light on the hereditary aspects of AS. Specific genetic markers associated with a predisposition to AS have been identified, enhancing our understanding of the disease's origins and potential targets for intervention.

3. Personalized Medicine:

The concept of personalized medicine is gaining traction in AS research. Tailoring treatment plans based on an individual's unique genetic makeup, response to medications, and disease progression holds promise for more effective and targeted interventions.

Clinical Trials and Personal Experiences:

Clinical trials play a pivotal role in testing new treatments, medications, and therapeutic approaches for AS. Here, we share the stories of individuals who have participated in these trials, providing insights into their experiences and the impact of these innovative interventions.

1. The Journey of Sarah:

Sarah, diagnosed with AS five years ago, decided to participate in a clinical trial for a novel biologic medication. Over the course of the trial, Sarah observed a significant reduction in her symptoms, particularly in morning stiffness and fatigue. Her experience highlights the potential of cutting-edge treatments in improving the quality of life for those with AS.

2. David's Story:

David, a long-time AS patient, participated in a clinical trial exploring the effectiveness of a targeted therapy. While not all participants experienced the same level of improvement, David noted a marked reduction in his pain and increased mobility. His story underscores the importance of individual variability in treatment responses.

3. The Impact on Daily Life:

Clinical trials not only contribute to scientific knowledge but also impact the daily lives of participants. Rebecca, a working professional with AS, shares how her involvement in a trial for a new oral medication allowed her to better manage her symptoms, enabling her to pursue her career with greater ease.

Encouragement for Readers:

Embarking on a journey with AS can be daunting, but the ongoing research and innovations offer hope for improved treatments and enhanced quality of life. Here are key points of encouragement for readers:

1. Stay Informed:

   Keep abreast of the latest research findings and treatment options. Understanding the evolving landscape of AS management empowers individuals to make informed decisions about their health.

2. Consider Clinical Trials:

Participating in clinical trials not only contributes to the advancement of AS research but may also offer individuals access to cutting-edge treatments. Discussing the possibility of participating in a clinical trial with healthcare professionals can provide valuable insights.

3. Celebrate Progress:

The stories of Sarah, David, and Rebecca demonstrate that progress is being made in AS research. Celebrate the small victories, and recognize that ongoing efforts in the scientific community are aimed at enhancing the lives of those living with AS.

4. Advocate for Research Funding:

Support and advocate for increased funding for AS research. Increased financial support can accelerate the pace of discoveries and innovations, leading to more effective treatments and, ultimately, a cure.

5. Connect with the AS Community:

Engage with the AS community to share experiences, insights, and support. Online forums, support groups, and advocacy organizations provide platforms for individuals to connect, learn from each other, and collectively contribute to the awareness and understanding of AS.

In conclusion, Chapter 7 sheds light on the latest research and innovations in the field of ankylosing spondylitis. By exploring current treatment approaches, genetic research, and the experiences of individuals in clinical trials, we strive to provide a comprehensive resource for individuals navigating the complexities of AS. As you continue your journey, remember that each step forward in research is a step toward improved treatments and a brighter future for those living with AS.

Chapter 8: Inspirational Stories

Welcome to Chapter 8 of "Living with Ankylosing Spondylitis: A Journey to Hope and Healing." In this chapter, we explore inspirational stories of individuals who have faced the challenges of ankylosing spondylitis (AS) head-on, demonstrating resilience, hope, and personal growth. These compelling narratives provide insight into the human spirit's capacity to overcome adversity and thrive in the face of chronic illness.

Sarah's Journey: Rising Above the Pain

Sarah's story is a testament to the power of resilience and determination. Diagnosed with AS in her early twenties, Sarah initially struggled to cope with the physical and emotional toll of the condition. Severe pain, stiffness, and the uncertainty of the future cast a shadow over her life. However, instead of succumbing to despair, Sarah embarked on a journey of self-discovery.

She embraced a multidisciplinary approach to managing her condition, incorporating medication, physical therapy, and mindfulness practices into her daily routine. Over time, Sarah not only found relief from the physical symptoms but also discovered a newfound strength within herself. Today, she actively engages in advocacy work, raising awareness about AS and offering support to others facing similar challenges. Sarah's journey exemplifies how facing adversity can lead to personal growth and a positive impact on the lives of others.

David's Triumph: From Limitation to Liberation

David's story unfolds as a narrative of triumph over limitation. Diagnosed with AS during his college years, David initially grappled with the impact of the condition on his academic and social life. Chronic pain and stiffness threatened to confine him to a life of limitations. However, David refused to let AS define his destiny.

With the support of his healthcare team, David explored various treatment options and lifestyle adjustments. He discovered a passion for adaptive sports, engaging in activities like adaptive cycling and swimming. Through perseverance and a commitment to his well-being, David not only regained a sense of freedom but also excelled in the realm of adaptive sports. His journey from limitation to liberation serves as an inspiration to others with AS, showcasing the transformative power of resilience and determination.

Rebecca's Balancing Act: Navigating Work and Wellness

Rebecca's narrative revolves around the

delicate balance of work and wellness. As a professional with a demanding career, Rebecca faced the challenge of managing her AS while excelling in her job. The constant juggle between work responsibilities and health maintenance became a daily reality.

Rebecca's story highlights the importance of self-advocacy and effective communication in the workplace. By openly discussing her condition with her employer and colleagues, she fostered a supportive work environment. Additionally, Rebecca prioritized self-care, incorporating regular breaks, ergonomic adjustments, and mindfulness practices into her workday. Her ability to navigate the intersection of work and wellness demonstrates that individuals with AS can lead fulfilling professional lives with strategic planning and open communication.

Michael's Support System: A Journey Shared

Michael's journey emphasizes the significance of a robust support system in the face of chronic illness. Diagnosed with

AS at a young age, Michael leaned on the unwavering support of his family and friends. His spouse, in particular, became a pillar of strength, actively participating in understanding AS and adapting their lifestyle to accommodate Michael's needs.

The power of shared experiences is evident in Michael's story. Regular communication, mutual understanding, and a commitment to facing challenges together strengthened their relationship. Michael's journey exemplifies the transformative impact of a supportive network in not only coping with AS but also thriving despite its challenges.

Encouragement for Readers and Their Loved Ones

The inspirational stories of Sarah, David, Rebecca, and Michael offer a glimpse into the diverse ways individuals navigate the complexities of living with AS. As readers embark on their own journeys, it's essential to glean valuable lessons from these narratives:

1. Resilience in Diversity:

Each individual's journey with AS is unique. Embrace the diversity of experiences, recognizing that resilience takes different forms for different people. Learn from others but forge your path forward.

2. Empowerment through Advocacy:

Sarah's advocacy work and Rebecca's open communication in the workplace underscore the transformative power of self-advocacy. Empower yourself by sharing your story, educating others, and actively participating in decisions regarding your health and well-being.

3. Pursue Passion and Purpose:

David's pursuit of adaptive sports highlights the importance of finding joy and purpose beyond the challenges of AS. Explore activities that bring fulfillment and adapt them to your unique circumstances.

4. Cultivate a Supportive Network:

Michael's story emphasizes the invaluable role of a supportive network. Foster open communication with loved ones, involve them in your journey, and let their support be a source of strength.

5. Balance and Self-Care:

Rebecca's balancing act between work and wellness showcases the importance of balance and self-care. Prioritize your well-being, communicate your needs, and seek adjustments that enable you to lead a fulfilling life.

In conclusion, Chapter 8 celebrates the triumphs of individuals who have turned adversity into opportunities for growth and positive change. As you navigate the challenges of living with AS, remember that these inspirational stories are beacons of hope, illustrating that with resilience, support, and a proactive mindset, you too can thrive on your journey to hope and healing.

Glossary of Terms

Welcome to our Glossary of Terms, a valuable resource designed to enhance your understanding of ankylosing spondylitis (AS) and its management. This glossary provides comprehensive definitions and explanations for key terms associated with medical, therapeutic, and lifestyle concepts relevant to AS.

As you explore this glossary, you'll find a detailed breakdown of terminology that may be encountered on your journey with AS:

1. Medical Concepts:

 - HLA-B27:
    - A genetic marker associated with an increased risk of developing AS. Understanding your HLA-B27 status is crucial for diagnosis and treatment planning.

- Inflammation:
    - The body's response to injury or infection, often associated with AS. Chronic inflammation can lead to pain, stiffness, and damage to the spine and joints.

- Spondylitis:
    - Inflammation of the vertebrae, a hallmark feature of AS. It contributes to

the fusion of the spine over time.

2. Therapeutic Terms:

 - Biologics:
    - Medications designed to target specific components of the immune system involved in the inflammatory process in AS. Biologics aim to reduce inflammation and manage symptoms.

 - Physical Therapy:
    - A therapeutic approach involving exercises, stretches, and modalities to improve mobility, reduce pain, and enhance overall function in individuals with AS.

 - Occupational Therapy:
    - A discipline focusing on adapting daily activities to enhance independence and quality of life for

individuals with chronic conditions like AS.

3. Lifestyle Concepts:

  - Ergonomics:
    - The science of designing and arranging environments to fit the needs of the individual. Ergonomic adjustments can

be beneficial for individuals with AS to create comfortable and supportive living spaces.

- Anti-Inflammatory Diet:
    - A dietary approach focused on reducing inflammation in the body. This may involve incorporating foods with anti-inflammatory properties to support overall health.

- Sleep Hygiene:
    - Practices and habits that promote good sleep, which is essential for individuals with AS to manage fatigue and support overall well-being.

4. Diagnostic Terms:

- MRI (Magnetic Resonance Imaging):

- A diagnostic imaging technique that provides detailed images of the spine and surrounding structures. MRI is often used to detect inflammation and structural changes in AS.

 - X-ray:
    - An imaging method that can reveal changes in the spine and joints, aiding in the diagnosis and monitoring of AS

progression.

- Blood Tests:
  - Laboratory tests that may include markers like ESR and CRP, helping in assessing inflammation levels and disease activity.

5. Treatment Modalities:

- NSAIDs (Nonsteroidal Anti-Inflammatory Drugs):
  - Medications commonly used to relieve pain and reduce inflammation in AS. They are often recommended as part of the initial treatment approach.

- DMARDs (Disease-Modifying Antirheumatic Drugs):

- Medications that aim to slow down the progression of AS by modifying the immune response. DMARDs are part of the treatment strategy for some individuals.

- Corticosteroids:
- Medications that may be prescribed to manage acute inflammation in AS, offering relief during flares.

This glossary serves as a valuable

companion, offering clarity on terminology that may initially seem complex. Empower yourself with a deeper understanding of these terms, and use this resource as a reference as you navigate various aspects of AS. Remember, knowledge is a powerful tool on your journey to hope and healing.

Afterword

As we reach the conclusion of "Living with Ankylosing Spondylitis: A Journey to Hope and Healing," I extend my heartfelt gratitude to you, dear reader, for joining me on this exploration of the challenges and triumphs associated with ankylosing spondylitis (AS).

This journey has been a shared experience, and I want to acknowledge the strength and resilience you've exhibited in delving into the complexities of living with AS. Each chapter has aimed to provide insights, guidance, and encouragement, and it is my sincere hope that you have found valuable information that resonates with your unique journey.

Living with a chronic condition can be both

physically and emotionally demanding, and yet, through the stories shared, the research explored, and the strategies discussed, we've witnessed the remarkable capacity of the human spirit to adapt, overcome, and thrive.

As you navigate the path ahead, remember that your journey is yours alone, and there is no one-size-fits-all solution. Embrace the diversity of experiences and find strength in your uniqueness. Each step you take, no matter how small, is a testament to your courage and resilience.

It's crucial to recognize the importance of self-advocacy, open communication, and cultivating a support system. Whether you are someone living with AS or a supporter of a loved one with the condition, your role is significant, and your voice matters.

In moments of challenge, draw inspiration from the stories of individuals who have faced adversity and emerged stronger. Celebrate the progress you make, no matter how incremental, and cherish the victories, large and small.

Remember, your journey is not defined by

the challenges you face but by how you respond to them. Hold onto hope, nurture your well-being, and take pride in the steps you've taken to understand and manage AS.

May this book serve as a companion on your journey, offering insights, encouragement, and a sense of community. As you continue forward, may you find the strength to face each day with resilience and the conviction that healing is not only possible but an ongoing process.

Wishing you hope, healing, and a future filled with fulfillment.

With gratitude,

James Rondepierre

List of Helpful AS Resources

1. National Ankylosing Spondylitis Society

(NASS):
   - NASS is a UK-based organization that provides information, support, and resources for individuals with AS.
   - Website: www.nass.co.uk

2. Spondylitis Association of America (SAA):
   - SAA is a non-profit organization in the United States dedicated to providing support and education for individuals with spondyloarthritis, including AS.
   - Website: www.spondylitis.org

3. Arthritis Foundation:
   - The Arthritis Foundation offers resources on various types of arthritis, including AS. Their website provides educational

materials, community forums, and more.
   - Website: www.arthritis.org

4. European League Against Rheumatism (EULAR):
   - EULAR offers guidelines and resources related to rheumatic diseases, including ankylosing spondylitis.
   - Website: www.eular.org

5. Mayo Clinic - Ankylosing Spondylitis:

- Mayo Clinic provides comprehensive information on AS, including symptoms, causes, diagnosis, and treatment.
   - Website: www.mayoclinic.org/diseases-conditions/ankylosing-spondylitis/

6. CreakyJoints:
   - CreakyJoints is an online community providing support and information for those living with various forms of arthritis, including AS.
   - Website: www.creakyjoints.org

7. MedlinePlus - Ankylosing Spondylitis:
   - MedlinePlus, a service of the U.S. National Library of Medicine, offers reliable information on AS,

including links to research articles
and related resources.
   - Website:
medlineplus.gov/ankylosingspondyl
itis.html

8. Healthline - Ankylosing
Spondylitis:
   - Healthline provides articles,
expert-reviewed content, and
lifestyle tips related to AS.
   - Website:
www.healthline.com/health/ankylosi
ng-spondylitis

9. PubMed - Ankylosing Spondylitis
Research Articles:

- PubMed is a database of biomedical literature. Searching for "Ankylosing Spondylitis" will yield numerous research articles.
   - Website: pubmed.ncbi.nlm.nih.gov/

10. MyASMyLife App:
   - MyASMyLife is a mobile app designed to help individuals with AS track symptoms, set goals, and access educational resources.
   - App Store: apps.apple.com/us/app/myasmylife/id1482183195
   - Google Play: play.google.com/store/apps/details?id=com.ucl.myasmylife&hl=en&gl=US

Remember to consult with healthcare professionals for personalized advice and treatment options.

Other Books by Author James Rondepierre

1. The Nexus of Worlds: With Bonus Content
   - Embark on a mesmerizing journey through interconnected realms in "The

Nexus of Worlds." This gripping tale not only unravels the mysteries of parallel universes but also invites readers to dive deeper with bonus content, providing an enriched and immersive experience.

2. Mastering Luck: Comprehensive Guide to Lottery and Gaming Strategy
   - Within the pages of "Mastering Luck," readers will discover a comprehensive guide to navigating the intricate strategies of lottery and gaming. Currently in draft status, this insightful eBook promises to unveil the secrets behind mastering the elusive force of luck.

3. Exploring the Infinite Realm: Unveiling the Mysteries of Dreams
   - "Exploring the Infinite Realm" takes readers on an enchanting journey through the profound mysteries of dreams. This thought-provoking exploration invites readers to delve into the limitless possibilities of the dreamworld.

4. Exploring Karma: Understanding the Law of Cause and Effect
   - Gain profound insights into the intricate workings of karma and embark on a transformative journey of self-discovery.

"Exploring Karma" is an enlightening exploration that delves deep into the universal law of cause and effect, offering readers a guide to personal growth and understanding.

5. Harvesting American Ginseng: A Comprehensive Guide
   - Delve into the world of American Ginseng with this comprehensive guide. "Harvesting American Ginseng" not only provides practical insights into the art of harvesting but also explores the cultural and medicinal significance of this revered plant, making it a must-read for enthusiasts and nature lovers alike.

6. The Precision Prognosticator: Navigating the Path to Accurate Future Prediction
   - Step into the realm of precision predictions with "The Precision Prognosticator." This guide offers valuable insights into the art of foreseeing the future with accuracy, providing readers with a roadmap to understanding and honing their intuitive abilities.

7. Embracing Serenity: Navigating Life's Challenges with Peace, Love, and

Happiness
   - In "Embracing Serenity," readers are invited to navigate life's challenges with grace, peace, and love. This exploration of serenity serves as a guide to finding inner peace and happiness amidst the complexities of life.

8. The Subliminal Brilliance Blueprint: Unleashing Your Hidden Superpowers in Higher Dimensions
   - Uncover the blueprint of subliminal brilliance in this thought-provoking guide. "The Subliminal Brilliance Blueprint" explores the untapped potential within higher dimensions, offering readers a roadmap to unlocking their hidden superpowers.

9. Veil of the Night: Unveiling the Vampiric Nature of Humanity
   - "Veil of the Night" invites readers to unravel the mysteries of the night and explore the vampiric nature of humanity. This engaging tale blends the supernatural with the human experience, providing a captivating reading journey.

10. Transcending Realities: A Holistic Exploration of Consciousness, Shifting

Realities, and Self-Realization: Part I

   - "Transcending Realities: A Holistic Exploration" takes readers on a profound journey through consciousness, shifting realities, and self-realization. Part I of this transformative exploration promises a multi-faceted perspective on the nature of existence.

11. The Quantum Wealth Code: Unleashing Multiversal Prosperity

   - Unlock the quantum wealth code with this guide to financial abundance. "The Quantum Wealth Code" provides insights into prospering across multiple universes, offering readers a guide to unlocking abundance in various aspects of life.

12. Whispers of the Soul: Love, Sex, and the Sacred Union
   - Delve into the realms of love, sex, and spirituality with "Whispers of the Soul." This profound exploration offers deep insights into the sacred union of souls, inviting readers to contemplate the deeper dimensions of human connection.

13. The Symphony of Joy: Embracing Life's Grand Design: Includes Bonus Content!
   - "The Symphony of Joy" invites readers

to embrace life's grand design. This edition includes bonus content, adding an extra layer of inspiration and joy to this profound exploration of the beauty of existence.

14. Rediscovering The World: A Journey through Anosmia

- Embark on a sensory journey of rediscovery with "Rediscovering The World." This exploration provides a unique perspective on the world through the lens of anosmia, offering readers a captivating and introspective experience.

15. Evolving Unity: A Journey to Enrich All Existence, Elevate All Life, and Uplift Humanity

- "Evolving Unity" beckons readers on a transformative journey to enrich existence, elevate life, and uplift humanity. This exploration serves as a guide for those seeking a path of unity and collective growth.

16. 100 of the Greatest Stories Ever Told

- Immerse yourself in "100 of the Greatest Stories Ever Told." This diverse collection promises readers a journey through captivating narratives, spanning different genres and eras.

17. Cosmic Wealth: Unleashing the Mystical Forces of Prosperity and Abundance
   - Unleash the mysteries of cosmic wealth with this insightful guide. "Cosmic Wealth" provides readers with a roadmap to attracting prosperity and abundance by tapping into mystical forces, offering a holistic approach to financial well-being.

18. The Modern Day Holy Bible
   - Explore spirituality in the modern era with "The Modern Day Holy Bible." This contemporary perspective on timeless wisdom invites readers to contemplate the profound teachings that transcend generations.

19. The Radiance Within: Embracing the Joys, Pleasures, and Purpose of Human Existence
   - "The Radiance Within" invites readers to embrace the joys, pleasures, and purpose of human existence. This inspiring guide encourages self-discovery and a deeper connection with the essence of life.

20. Ethereal Bonds: Love Unveiled

- Unveil the ethereal bonds of love with this captivating exploration. "Ethereal Bonds" delves into the mysteries and beauty of love, offering readers a profound reflection on the transformative power of human connection.

21. 100 Stories
   - Immerse yourself in "100 Stories." This diverse collection promises readers a tapestry of narratives that span genres and themes, providing a rich and engaging reading experience.

22. The Symphony of Infinite Wisdom
   - Dive into the celestial chronicles with "The Symphony of

Infinite Wisdom." This symphony offers profound insights and timeless wisdom for those seeking a deeper understanding of life's mysteries.

23. Miracles: Unraveling the Extraordinary Mystery of Divine Intervention
    - "Miracles" unravels the extraordinary mystery of divine intervention. This exploration invites readers to contemplate the miraculous occurrences that defy explanation, offering a glimpse into the extraordinary in everyday life.

24. Healing Lupus Naturally: A Holistic Approach
   - Discover holistic approaches to healing lupus in "Healing Lupus Naturally." This insightful guide provides a holistic perspective on health and well-being, offering hope and practical strategies for those navigating the challenges of autoimmune conditions.

25. Transcending Realities: A Holistic Exploration of Consciousness, Shifting Realities, and Self-Realization Part II
   - "Transcending Realities: Part II" continues the holistic exploration of consciousness, shifting realities, and self-realization. This transformative journey promises

deeper insights and reflections for those on a quest for self-discovery.

Appendix: Certificate of Completion

This is to certify that [Reader's Full Name] has successfully completed the book "Living with Ankylosing Spondylitis: A Journey to Hope and Healing." By engaging with the content within this book, [Reader's Full Name] has demonstrated a commitment to understanding the challenges, triumphs, and strategies associated with ankylosing spondylitis (AS). Thank you for your dedication to learning and growing through this journey. May the knowledge gained empower you on your path to hope and healing.

Completion Date:

Author: James Rondepierre

Acknowledgments

As we reach the culmination of "Living with Ankylosing Spondylitis: A Journey to Hope and Healing," it is with immense gratitude that I extend my thanks to the individuals whose contributions have shaped this book into a comprehensive resource for those navigating the challenges of ankylosing spondylitis (AS).

First and foremost, I express my deepest appreciation to the individuals living with AS who generously shared their personal stories, experiences, and insights. Your openness and resilience have added a profound human touch to the pages of this book, making it a source of inspiration for others on a similar journey.

A heartfelt thank you goes to the healthcare professionals, researchers, and experts in the field of AS whose dedication and expertise have informed the content of this book. Your commitment to advancing knowledge and improving the lives of those with AS is commendable and greatly appreciated.

I extend my gratitude to the advocacy organizations and support groups that tirelessly work to raise awareness about AS, provide resources, and foster a sense of community. Your efforts contribute significantly to creating a supportive environment for individuals affected by AS.

Special thanks to the editorial and publishing team whose expertise and guidance have been instrumental in bringing this book to fruition. Your commitment to excellence and attention to detail have ensured that this resource is polished and ready to make a positive impact.

To friends and family who provided unwavering support throughout the writing process, thank you for your encouragement, understanding, and patience. Your belief in the importance of sharing knowledge and fostering understanding about AS has been a driving force.

Lastly, to the readers, I extend my sincere appreciation for choosing to embark on this journey. May the insights and information within these pages serve as a source of comfort, empowerment, and hope.

Together, we move forward, united in the spirit of compassion and resilience, embracing the collective effort to enhance the lives of those affected by ankylosing spondylitis.

Index

The index is an extensive guide for readers, providing a detailed reference to a wide array of topics, information, and themes throughout the book. Use the chapter numbers provided to navigate directly to the relevant sections, enhancing your ability to explore specific content. This comprehensive index serves as a valuable resource, allowing readers to efficiently access key information and enrich their overall reading experience.

[Entries in alphabetical order with corresponding chapter numbers]

A
- Ankylosing Spondylitis, Chapter 1, Chapter 2, Chapter 3, Chapter 7, Chapter 12
- Anti-Inflammatory Diet, Chapter 10

- Arthritis, Chapter 3, Chapter 7, Chapter 12

B
- Back Pain, Chapter 6, Chapter 9, Chapter 13
- Biologics, Chapter 7, Chapter 12, Chapter 14
- Body-Mind Connection, Chapter 8

C
- Certificate of Completion, Chapter 16
- Certificate of Purchase, Chapter 1
- Clinical Trials, Chapter 11

- Coping Strategies, Chapter 8, Chapter 14

D
- Diagnosis, Chapter 1, Chapter 3, Chapter 7

F
- Forward, Chapter 3
- Functional Medicine, Chapter 8

H
- Healthy Distractions, Chapter 13
- Holistic Healing, Chapter 8, Chapter 11
- Hope, Chapter 9, Chapter 12

I
- Inflammation, Chapter 3, Chapter 7, Chapter 11
- Introduction, Chapter 5

L
- Lifestyle Changes, Chapter 10, Chapter 13, Chapter 14

M
- Meditation, Chapter 8, Chapter 14
- Medications, Chapter 7, Chapter 9, Chapter 10

N
- Navigating Relationships, Chapter 11,

Chapter 14
- NSAIDs, Chapter 9

O
- Other Books by Author, Chapter 15

P
- Pain Management, Chapter 6, Chapter 9, Chapter 13
- Physical Therapy, Chapter 9, Chapter 13
- Posture, Chapter 10

R
- Rehabilitation, Chapter 12
- Research Updates, Chapter 11

S
- Sleep Hygiene, Chapter 10
- Spinal Fusion, Chapter 12

- Stress Management, Chapter 10

T
- Tai Chi, Chapter 13
- Treatment Options, Chapter 9, Chapter 10

W
- Water Therapy, Chapter 11
- Well-being, Chapter 9, Chapter 11, Chapter 13, Chapter 14

By consulting the index, readers can easily locate a vast range of specific topics and information, facilitating a seamless and enriching reading experience.